FROM MANAGING TO CONQUERING DIFFICULT SWALLOWING

Expert guide to Understanding the Causes, Recognizing Symptoms, and Embracing Effective Treatments for a Life of Health and Vitality

DR. DASHIELL DANIEL

The book "Difficult Swallowing" distinguishes itself as a thorough manual in the dysphagia field and becomes a valuable tool for researchers, medical professionals, and people who are interested in or experiencing the difficulties of swallowing disorders. The methodical examination of the anatomical, neurological, and functional facets of the swallowing mechanism in Chapter 1 of this publication highlights its multidimensional nature and offers a sophisticated understanding of the normal swallowing process. In Chapter 2, the book explores the complexities of the causes of problematic swallowing, from neurological illnesses to structural deformities. This makes the book an invaluable resource for diagnosing and contextualizing a wide range of etiologies.

The importance of 'Difficult Swallowing' goes beyond identification, since Chapter 3 delves deeply into the symptoms and diagnostic approaches, utilizing cutting-edge methods like video fluoroscopy and endoscopic assessment. Chapter 4 presents a wide range of therapy methods that not only assist healthcare professionals but also provide empowerment to persons who are experiencing issues with swallowing. These interventions range from rehabilitative activities to surgical interventions. Moreover, Chapters 5 and 6's inclusion of coping mechanisms and lifestyle adjustments enhances the book by offering helpful advice on how to handle and lessen the psychological effects of dysphagia.

The proactive approach adopted in Chapter 7, which clarifies preventive techniques and emphasizes the need for early diagnosis and action, is noteworthy. The book positions itself as an ally in fostering holistic well-being by going beyond its role as a simple clinical reference and including preventive strategies, lifestyle guidelines, and support systems.

To summarize, 'Difficult Swallowing' is a comprehensive resource that offers insightful guidance to scholars and professionals alike, combines cutting-edge research with real-world applications, and makes a substantial contribution to the conversation around dysphagia."

Introduction

Dysphagia, the medical term for difficulty swallowing, is a multifaceted and complex condition that affects a large percentage of the population. It is characterized by disruptions in the normal swallowing process, which includes the complex coordination of muscles and nerves involved in moving food and liquids from the mouth to the stomach.

Dysphagia can present at any stage of life, causing problems ranging from mild discomfort to severe complications that have an impact on both physical and psychological well-being.

Since swallowing is a necessary function for maintaining life, any difficulty swallowing should be thoroughly investigated and comprehended.

The Objective Of The Book

With a focus on the etiology, diagnosis, and management of dysphagia, this book aims to bridge the gap between clinical knowledge and public awareness by offering a thorough exploration of the complex aspects of difficult swallowing. It is an essential resource for healthcare professionals, including physicians, speech-language pathologists, nurses, and researchers, who are seeking a thorough understanding of dysphagia. Additionally, the book empowers individuals who are struggling with swallowing difficulties by promoting self-advocacy and educating them to make informed decisions about their health.

The Intended Audience

This book is intended for a wide range of readers with differing degrees of experience in the healthcare field. It primarily serves the needs of medical students, clinicians, and therapists, providing a thorough overview of dysphagia that combines theoretical understanding with practical application. It is also meant to be used by people outside of the healthcare field, such as patients, caregivers, and anyone who wants to learn more about the difficulties involved in difficult swallowing. By adapting the content to different levels of expertise, this book hopes to foster cooperation and understanding among diverse stakeholders in the dysphagia field.

Synopsis Of Troublesome Swallowing

The term dysphagia refers to a range of difficulties associated with the oral, pharyngeal, and oesophageal phases of swallowing.

The oral phase entails chewing and creating a cohesive bolus; the pharyngeal phase is critical for initiating the swallowing reflex and preventing aspiration; and the oesophageal phase involves the passage of the bolus through the esophagus into the stomach.

There are numerous causes of dysphagia, including neurological disorders, structural abnormalities, and functional impairments. Common etiologist include stroke, neurodegenerative diseases, head and neck cancers, and muscular disorders. Diagnosis frequently entails a combination of clinical assessment, imaging tests, and endoscopic procedures to identify the cause of the problem.

A multidisciplinary approach is necessary for the effective management of dysphagia, involving the collaboration of physicians, speech-language pathologists, dietitians, and other allied health professionals. Depending on the type and severity of the swallowing impairment, treatment modalities range from dietary modifications and rehabilitative exercises to surgical interventions. The psychological impact of dysphagia is significant, and this book addresses the psychosocial aspects of living with difficult swallowing, addressing the difficulties that individuals face and offering coping strategies and strategies for improving quality of life.

By providing a thorough overview, this book aims to advance the understanding of difficult swallowing across multiple dimensions, promoting a holistic approach.

CHAPTER ONE
A COMPREHENSIVE GLOBAL VIEW

The anatomy of the swallowing mechanism is a complex interaction of different structures and functions that allow food to pass easily from the mouth to the stomach. During the oral phase, food is manipulated and formed into a cohesive bolus that can be swallowed. Saliva, which is full of enzymes, helps break down carbohydrates at the beginning of the process, which makes the subsequent stages of digestion easier.

The oral phase is important for both mechanical breakdown and sensory feedback, which lets the person know what the food is like.

The oral phase is followed by the pharyngeal phase, which is the change from voluntary to involuntary control. The upper oesophageal sphincter relaxes, allowing the bolus to enter the esophagus, and problems like aspiration pneumonia can arise when the protective mechanisms are not functioning properly.

The coordinated movements of the soft palate, pharynx, and larynx guarantee the appropriate closure of the airway to prevent food aspiration into the respiratory system.

The last phase of swallowing is known as the oesophageal phase, and it is characterized by the peristaltic movement of the esophagus, which pushes food particles toward the stomach.

The lower oesophageal sphincter is essential in preventing reflux of stomach contents into the esophagus, which keeps the digestive process intact. Disturbances that impact the oesophageal phase can result in regurgitation, discomfort, and even more serious complications like esophagitis.

The complex process of swallowing is controlled by the integration of the central and peripheral nervous systems. The brainstem, in particular the medulla and pons, is involved in the coordination of the different stages of swallowing.

The brain receives feedback from sensory receptors in the oral cavity and pharynx, which enables adjustments in the swallowing process. Neurological disorders, such as degenerative diseases or strokes, can have a significant impact on swallowing function by causing disruptions to the complex neural pathways that control this essential physiological function.

When analyzing the normal swallowing process, it is critical to recognize the dynamic interaction between anatomy and neurology.

Achieving a successful swallow requires the smooth synchronization of muscle contractions, accurate timing, and efficient sensory feedback. Combining these components guarantees the effective passage of food particles to the stomach while protecting the airway from any complications. Recognizing and treating abnormalities related to the normal swallowing process lays the groundwork for promoting optimal nutrition and general health.

Having Trouble Swallowing

Dysphagia is the term for the presentation of swallowing difficulties that can result from a variety of causes and have a substantial negative influence on a person's quality of life. Dysphagia can be classified according to the phase of swallowing that is affected; oral, pharyngeal, and oesophageal dysphagia all pose different difficulties.

People who have oral dysphagia typically have problems with the early phases of swallowing, which are mainly related to mastication and the creation of a cohesive bolus. Oral motor disorders, neuromuscular deficits, or poor dentition can all be contributing factors to oral dysphagia.

People who have oral dysphagia may also have trouble manipulating food in the mouth, which can result in longer meal times, less food intake, and nutritional deficiencies.

Conversely, pharyngeal dysphagia refers to problems with the involuntary phase of swallowing.

Incomplete closure of the airway due to poor coordination of the pharyngeal phase muscles increases the risk of aspiration. Pharyngeal dysphagia may be caused by neurological disorders, anatomical abnormalities, or weakening of the muscles. To minimize complications, pharyngeal dysphagia requires careful assessment and focused interventions.

Disorders affecting the lower oesophageal sphincter, such as achalasia or gastroesophageal reflux disease (GERD), may also contribute to oesophageal dysphagia. The symptoms of oesophageal dysphagia are challenges in the final stage of swallowing, often involving a sensation of food sticking or difficulty in passing the bolus through the esophagus. Structural abnormalities, such as strictures or tumors, can impede the smooth flow of ingested material.

Understanding the specific neurological underpinnings of dysphagia is crucial for developing targeted rehabilitation strategies and optimizing outcomes for affected individuals.

Dysphagia is closely linked to the neurological control of swallowing because disruptions in the neural pathways governing this process can result in significant functional impairments. Neurological conditions such as stroke, traumatic brain injury, or neurodegenerative diseases like Parkinson's disease can compromise the intricate coordination required for effective swallowing.

The normal swallowing process is disrupted when someone has dysphagia; therefore, a thorough assessment is necessary to determine the underlying cause and modify interventions appropriately. Dysphagia affects more than just the ability to swallow; it also affects respiratory health, nutritional status, and general well-being. Healthcare professionals—such as speech-language pathologists, neurologists, and gastroenterologists—must work together to manage dysphagia holistically, addressing both its symptomatic manifestations and underlying causes.

Clinical Assessment Of Troubles With Swallowing

An extensive assessment of the anatomical, physiological, and neurological aspects of the swallowing mechanism is part of the meticulous clinical evaluation of dysphagia. A detailed understanding of the patient's medical history, including any pre-existing conditions, medications, and previous interventions, forms the basis for a targeted evaluation.

Patient interviews are used to collect subjective data in the first phase of the evaluation.

Questions are asked about the symptoms that patients experience, such as food sticking, pain when swallowing, regurgitation, or coughing during or after meals. It is important to investigate the frequency, timing, and aggravating or mitigating factors of these symptoms.

Patient-reported outcomes, like weight loss or changes in dietary preferences, provide important information about how dysphagia affects daily life.

The clinical evaluation of dysphagia is greatly aided by objective assessment techniques.

Two commonly used imaging modalities that provide real-time visualization of the swallowing process are fibreoptic endoscopic evaluation of swallowing (FEES) and video fluoroscopic swallowing study (VFSS). FEES involve inserting a flexible endoscope through the nasal passages to directly observe the swallowing structures, providing valuable information about the coordination of movements, presence of aspiration, and structural abnormalities. VFSS, on the other hand, uses fluoroscopy to capture dynamic images of the swallowing process, allowing for the assessment of bolus transit, airway protection, and oesophageal function.

Apart from imaging studies, objective measurements such as manometry, which measures variations in oesophageal pressure and evaluates the function of the lower oesophageal sphincter, and electromyography (EMG), which measures the electrical activity of the swallowing muscles and provides information on neuromuscular coordination, can be used in conjunction with imaging studies to further improve the accuracy of the diagnostic process.

Understanding dysphagia requires a thorough understanding of neurological evaluation, especially when taking into account the effects of conditions like stroke, traumatic brain injury, or neurodegenerative diseases.

Clinical examination of cranial nerves, reflex assessment, and motor and sensory function evaluation all contribute to the patient's neurological profile. Working with neurologists and other specialists is frequently required to incorporate the results of neurological assessments into the overall treatment plan.

A comprehensive approach that takes into account the wider effects of swallowing difficulties on the patient's quality of life is involved in the clinical evaluation of dysphagia, which goes beyond the identification of structural or functional abnormalities. Nutritionists may be consulted to address any nutritional deficiencies resulting from dysphagia, and speech-language pathologists are essential in the design of therapeutic interventions to improve swallowing function.

To sum up, the clinical assessment of swallowing difficulties is a multifaceted procedure that blends subjective and objective evaluations to obtain a thorough grasp of the fundamental elements causing dysphagia. This coordinated strategy enables focused interventions, varying from therapeutic activities to pharmaceutical or surgical procedures, with the ultimate aim of restoring swallowing ability and augmenting the general welfare of those impacted by dysphagia.

Handling Swallowing Challenges

Dysphagia management is a multidisciplinary, team-based process that includes therapeutic interventions, dietary changes, and, in certain situations, medical or surgical approaches.

It is important to customize the management plan based on the individual's severity of dysphagia and the underlying causes to maximize results and enhance the quality of life for those who are affected.

Rehabilitative strategies that aim to improve swallowing function are a key component of managing dysphagia. Speech-language pathologists are key players in this process, using exercises that focus on the strength and coordination of the swallowing muscles, such as tongue exercises, thermal-tactile stimulation, and maneuvers to improve the coordination of the oral and pharyngeal phases of swallowing. The ultimate goal of rehabilitation is to promote safer and more efficient swallowing, lowering the risk of complications like aspiration.

When neurological conditions like stroke or Parkinson's disease are the primary cause of dysphagia, a multidisciplinary approach is necessary.

Physical and occupational therapy as well as neurorehabilitation address the broader motor and functional deficits that underlie dysphagia. Adaptive techniques, like changing the consistency of food or positioning the body during meals, can be used to improve safety and the overall eating experience.

Texture-modified diets, such as pureed or thickened liquids, may be recommended to reduce the risk of aspiration. Speech-language pathologists and dietitians collaborate to develop personalized dietary plans that balance nutritional requirements with the individual's ability to safely swallow. Education and training for caregivers are essential to ensuring consistent adherence to dietary recommendations. Dietary modifications are a key component of managing dysphagia, tailored to the specific needs and abilities of the individual.

Surgical interventions, such as fundoplication for GERD or myotomy for achalasia, may be recommended in certain cases, especially when conservative measures prove insufficient.

In certain cases, medical interventions may be considered to address structural abnormalities contributing to dysphagia. Endoscopic procedures, such as dilation of esophageal strictures or the injection of botulinum toxin to treat conditions like achalasia, can be effective in restoring normal swallowing function.

In certain situations, such as when treating gastric acidity in GERD patients, pharmacological management may be used. However, the role of medications in managing dysphagia is typically supportive, and their efficacy is contingent upon the underlying cause of swallowing difficulties.

Beyond the clinical setting, dysphagia management emphasizes the value of continuous education and support for both the dysphagic person and their caregivers.

 Lifestyle changes, like mindful eating and pacing during meals, can enhance the eating experience. Follow-up evaluations are crucial to track progress, make necessary adjustments to interventions, and address any new issues that may arise.

the management of swallowing difficulties necessitates a thorough and customized approach that takes into account the unique etiology, severity, and impact on the individual's life. Collaboration between healthcare professionals— such as speech-language pathologists, dietitians, neurologists, and gastroenterologists—is crucial to the development and execution of a customized management plan. The management of dysphagia seeks to improve the overall health and quality of life for those who struggle with swallowing.

CHAPTER TWO

REASONS FOR HAVING DIFFICULTY FOLLOWING

Several underlying factors can cause dysphagia, or difficulty swallowing; these can be broadly classified into three categories: structural, neurological, and functional. Each category includes specific conditions that impair the ability to swallow normally. Diagnosing and treating dysphagic patients effectively depends on knowing the causes of their difficulties.

Structural Causes

Physical abnormalities in the oral and pharyngeal regions are a common cause of difficulty swallowing. One important factor in this category is tumors, which can press against the swallowing structures and cause disturbances to the coordinated movements needed to pass food and liquids. Other abnormalities in the mouth or throat, like strictures or malformations, can also obstruct the smooth passage of ingested material and result in dysphagia. Determining the nature and extent of these structural problems is essential to developing treatment plans that are appropriate for the particular obstruction.

Reasons Neurological

The regulation and coordination of swallowing are largely dependent on neurological factors. Dysphagia can arise from any disturbance of the complex neural pathways involved in this process. Stroke, a primary cause of neurological impairment, can damage the brain regions responsible for coordinating swallowing movements. Stroke victims may have trouble initiating and completing the swallowing reflex. Parkinson's Disease, which is characterized by progressive degeneration of dopaminergic neurons, can also cause dysphagia.

The loss of motor control in the swallowing muscles can result in inefficient or unsafe swallowing patterns. Amyotrophic Lateral

Sclerosis (ALS), a neurodegenerative disease, can also affect the motor neurons responsible for swallowing.

Reasonable Causes

The normal aging process and some medical conditions affecting the gastrointestinal tract are frequently linked to functional causes of difficulty swallowing. Dysphagia in aging is a complex phenomenon that can arise from age-related changes in muscle strength, coordination, and sensation. As people age, the muscles involved in swallowing may weaken, and the overall effectiveness of the swallowing process may decline. Another functional cause of dysphagia is Gastroesophageal reflux disease (GERD), which can result from chronic exposure of the esophagus to stomach acid, which can cause inflammation and scarring. These changes in the oesophageal mucosa can cause structural abnormalities that impede the smooth passage of food.

To sum up, there are many different and complex reasons why people have trouble swallowing, including structural, neurological, and functional factors. For medical professionals to make an accurate diagnosis and create customized treatment plans for each patient, they must have a thorough understanding of these underlying causes. Research on the subject is still ongoing and will help us understand dysphagia better, which will lead to more creative approaches to diagnosis, management, and rehabilitation.

CHAPTER THREE
DIAGNOSIS AND SYMPTOMS

The medical term dysphagia refers to a group of symptoms that typically appear in the oropharyngeal or oesophageal stages of the swallowing process. Common symptoms include feeling as though food is stuck in the throat or chest, coughing or choking during eating, experiencing unexplained weight loss, and recurring pneumonia that is caused by food or liquids getting into the airway. Diagnosing and treating dysphagia requires knowledge of these symptoms.

Typical Signs And Symptoms Of Trouble Swallowing

Depending on the underlying cause, the symptoms of difficulty swallowing can vary greatly.

For example, oesophageal dysphagia frequently presents as a feeling of food becoming lodged in the chest, while oropharyngeal dysphagia may present as difficulty initiating a swallow, leading to coughing or choking. Patients may also experience pain or discomfort during swallowing, which can lead to reduced oral intake and unintended weight loss. A thorough assessment is necessary to identify the precise type and cause of the dysphagia.

Procedures For Diagnosis

A precise diagnosis of dysphagia is essential for customized treatment regimens. A range of diagnostic techniques are utilized to evaluate the oropharyngeal and oesophageal phases of swallowing, guaranteeing a comprehensive comprehension of the underlying problems.

Fluoroscopic Videography

A modified barium swallow study, or video fluoroscopy, is a dynamic imaging modality that provides real-time X-ray images of the swallowing process.

Patients go through the procedure of consuming a barium contrast medium mixed with food and liquid of varying consistencies, and the radiologist watches as the barium moves through the esophagus and oropharynx, identifying any abnormalities in structure, motility, or aspiration events. Video fluoroscopy is a valuable tool for diagnosing oropharyngeal and oesophageal dysphagia, providing in-depth knowledge about the mechanics of swallowing.

Endoscopic Assessment

Endoscopic evaluation entails using flexible endoscopes to view the structures inside the upper gastrointestinal tract. When it comes to endoscopic evaluation for difficult swallowing, two main types of endoscopy are typically used: trans nasal esophagoscopy (TNE) and upper gastrointestinal endoscopy (esophagogastroduodenoscopy, or EGD). TNE is a less invasive procedure that provides a detailed view of the esophagus, which makes it especially useful for evaluating oropharyngeal dysphagia. Both types of endoscopy are essential for identifying structural lesions and evaluating mucosal integrity.

Manometry

When used in conjunction with other diagnostic modalities, oesophageal manometry improves the accuracy of dysphagia diagnosis and directs appropriate therapeutic interventions. Oesophageal manometry is a diagnostic procedure intended to evaluate the motility and pressure dynamics of the esophagus. It entails the insertion of a catheter with pressure sensors through the nose and into the esophagus. As the patient swallows, the sensors measure the strength and coordination of muscular contractions along the length of the esophagus.

To sum up, swallowing difficulties are a major source of difficulties for people, impacting their nutritional status, quality of life, and general health.

One of the most important ways to identify the underlying causes of dysphagia is to identify the common symptoms and use advanced diagnostic techniques like video fluoroscopy, endoscopic evaluation, and manometry. Developing individualized treatment plans that are based on functional assessments, clinical evaluations, and imaging studies requires a multidisciplinary approach. Research and advancements in diagnostic techniques will help us better understand the complexities of swallowing difficulties and provide effective interventions for better patient outcomes.

CHAPTER FOUR
POSSIBLE TREATMENTS
Exercises For Rehabilitation

The management of dysphagia, a condition characterized by difficulty swallowing, is greatly aided by the use of swallowing therapy, a subset of rehabilitation exercises. Swallowing therapy consists of specific exercises intended to increase the strength and coordination of the swallowing muscles. Speech-language pathologists frequently lead patients through customized regimens that improve the neuromuscular control required for effective swallowing. These exercises may include lip exercises, tongue exercises, and other maneuvers that reinforce the complex interactions between the muscles involved in swallowing.

Exercises for the tongue and throat are an essential part of dysphagia rehabilitation. They target the muscles of the tongue and throat, which are important for the beginning and development of the swallowing reflex.

These exercises can be classified as a range of motion exercises for the throat muscles, resistance exercises, or tongue protrusion exercises.

The goal of these targeted exercises is to improve the muscular strength and coordination needed for the complex series of movements involved in swallowing. Additionally, therapists frequently use biofeedback techniques to give patients immediate feedback about how their muscles are functioning.

Drugs

Medication is another important treatment option for dysphagia. For example, muscle relaxants are used to treat swallowing difficulties caused by overactive or spasmodic muscles; they function by reducing excessive muscle contractions, which facilitates smoother and more controlled swallowing. Nevertheless, the use of muscle relaxants must be carefully considered in light of potential side effects and the underlying cause of dysphagia to ensure appropriate and targeted intervention.

Another class of medications used to treat difficulty swallowing is proton pump inhibitors (PPIs). PPIs are usually linked to decreased gastric acid production. When acid reflux is a contributing factor to dysphagia, PPIs can lessen the damaging effects of stomach acid on the lining of the esophagus. By treating the underlying cause of dysphagia, PPIs add to the overall management strategy, particularly when gastroesophageal reflux disease (GERD) is involved.

Surgical Procedures

Surgical interventions are an effective treatment for difficult swallowing when non-surgical measures are not enough. Dilatation procedures, for instance, use balloons or dilators to mechanically widen the esophagus to relieve constriction or narrowing. This procedure stretches the affected area and returns it to its normal function. Dilatation procedures are especially helpful in cases where dysphagia is caused by conditions such as oesophageal strictures, in which the lumen is narrowed because of scarring or inflammation.

Structural repair is a more complex intervention that addresses anatomical abnormalities that contribute to dysphagia. Disorders like tumors or hiatal hernias may require surgical correction to restore the proper anatomical configuration of the esophagus. Surgical repair entails meticulous procedures to rectify structural anomalies, frequently involving the skills of thoracic surgeons or gastroenterologists. Thorough preoperative assessment and accurate diagnosis are crucial in determining the best surgical strategy for each patient's unique situation.

Dietary Adjustments

A key component of managing dysphagia is dietary modifications, which center on modifying food and liquid consistencies to promote safer swallowing. When a patient experiences swallowing difficulties, a speech-language pathologist may suggest modifications like changing food textures or fluid thickness to lower the risk of aspiration. Thickening agents can be added to liquids to make them easier to swallow for people with dysphagia and help prevent aspiration into the airways.

These modifications are usually based on a comprehensive evaluation of the patient's swallowing abilities and nutritional needs, guaranteeing a safe and well-balanced diet.

In summary, the complex nature of dysphagia requires a multimodal approach to treatment. Rehabilitation exercises, such as targeted muscle exercises and swallowing therapy, address the neuromuscular aspects of dysphagia.

Medications, such as muscle relaxants and proton pump inhibitors, provide pharmacological interventions to manage specific underlying causes.

Surgical interventions, such as structural repairs and dilatation procedures, become necessary when conservative measures are not effective.

Finally, dietary modifications are critical in adjusting nutritional intake to the patient's swallowing abilities. Ultimately, this multimodal approach, which frequently involves collaboration among multiple healthcare providers

CHAPTER FIVE
MODIFYING YOUR LIFESTYLE FOR BETTER SWALLOWING

Healthcare professionals often recommend an upright posture with the head slightly tilted forward, promoting a more direct and unobstructed passage for the bolus. Patients with dysphagia, or difficulty swallowing, should be educated on the importance of proper body alignment during meals. Appropriate positioning guarantees optimal coordination of the swallowing muscles and facilitates the safe passage of food and liquids through the digestive tract.

Techniques For Swallowing

Swallowing techniques encompass a range of strategies aimed at enhancing the efficiency and safety of the swallowing process. Therapists often collaborate with dysphagia patients to introduce specific maneuvers and exercises designed to strengthen the muscles involved in swallowing. One such technique is the Mendelsohn maneuver, which focuses on prolonging the elevation of the larynx during swallowing, promoting improved bolus transit. The effortful swallow technique is another approach that encourages patients to exert extra force during the swallow, aiding in the clearance of residues. These techniques are tailored to address the underlying causes of dysphagia, providing patients with practical skills to navigate swallowing challenges.

Nutritional Guidelines

Dietary guidelines are critical for ensuring adequate nutrition while reducing the risk of aspiration and choking. Physicians and dietitians work together to create customized meal plans that meet the unique requirements of each patient.

A lot of emphasis is placed on adjusting food textures to the individual's ability to swallow; soft, moist, and easily chewable foods are advised to lower the risk of blockage or aspiration.

Portion control and mindful eating are also encouraged to avoid overloading the impaired swallowing mechanism. Dietary guidelines address not only the kinds of foods but also their frequency and timing to maximize the eating experience.

Diets Modified By Texture

Texture-modified diets are an essential part of managing dysphagia and are the foundation of dietary guidelines for these patients.

Texture-modified diets involve modifying food textures to better suit the patient's swallowing abilities. Pureed, minced, or chopped textures are common modifications that provide options that are easier to manipulate and swallow.

The type of texture modification that is chosen depends on the patient's needs, taking into account factors like oral muscle strength and coordination. Texture-modified diets aim to balance nutritional adequacy with safety during swallowing, preventing complications like aspiration pneumonia.

Collaboration between speech-language pathologists, dietitians, and caregivers

Suggested Liquid Consistency

Recommendations for liquid consistency are important factors to take into account when managing difficult swallowing, as they deal with issues related to thin and thick fluids. People who have dysphagia may have trouble with liquids because they have trouble coordinating the oral and pharyngeal phases of swallowing.

To help with these issues, healthcare providers frequently suggest changes to liquid viscosity.

Thickened liquids—achieved by adding thickeners—can help slow down the flow of liquids, reducing the risk of aspiration. On the other hand, some patients may find thin liquids more manageable, so customized recommendations are required. It's important to strike a balance between keeping patients hydrated and guaranteeing safety during swallowing.

To sum up, lifestyle modifications that promote better swallowing involve a variety of positioning, swallowing techniques, and dietary adjustments. These strategies are carefully crafted to improve the safety and effectiveness of the swallowing process while meeting the specific requirements of those who have trouble swallowing. Putting these ideas into practice calls for cooperation between healthcare providers, speech therapists, dietitians, and caregivers to guarantee a comprehensive and individualized approach to managing dysphagia.

CHAPTER SIX
SUPPORT AND COPING METHODS

Dysphagia, or difficulty swallowing, can have a significant negative influence on a person's physical and emotional health.

Coping mechanisms, such as cognitive restructuring, mindfulness, and psychoeducation, are used to help individuals cope with the emotional challenges that arise from impaired swallowing function. From a psychological standpoint, it is important to understand the nature of dysphagia. Patients frequently experience feelings of frustration, anxiety, and even depression as a result of these limitations. Cognitive-behavioral therapy (CBT) is one therapeutic intervention that may be used to address negative thought patterns and encourage more adaptive coping mechanisms.

Resources And Support Groups

Support groups are an essential part of the comprehensive care of people who have trouble swallowing. They give patients a forum to discuss their struggles, triumphs, and strategies for managing dysphagia. Being a part of these groups helps people feel less alone because they promote a sense of community and understanding.

In addition, people with swallowing difficulties can benefit from practical insights into coping mechanisms, lifestyle adjustments, and information about resources. The professionals who lead these groups, like speech-language pathologists and psychologists, are crucial in facilitating discussions and offering evidence-based information. Finally, online forums and virtual support groups enhance accessibility, e.g.

Techniques Of Communication

Difficulty swallowing affects more than just the act of eating; it also has an impact on communication. When people have dysphagia, it can make it difficult for them to communicate clearly and to engage in general. To address these difficulties, different communication strategies are used to increase understanding and participation. Speech-language pathologists work with people who have dysphagia to create customized strategies that may involve changing speech rates, emphasizing certain sounds, or using alternative communication devices. These strategies are intended to increase communication efficiency and guarantee that people with dysphagia can express themselves and engage in social situations. In addition, teaching

Effects Of Difficulty Swallowing On The Mind

The psychological impact of difficult swallowing is multifaceted and extends beyond the physical challenges associated with dysphagia. Individuals grappling with swallowing difficulties often experience a range of emotions, including frustration, embarrassment, and a sense of loss of control. The inability to enjoy meals or share communal dining experiences may lead to feelings of isolation and depression. Furthermore, the fear of choking or aspiration can create anxiety and avoidance behaviors around eating. Psychologically, addressing these issues involves a comprehensive approach that combines psychoeducation, counseling, and, in some cases, pharmacological interventions. Tailoring interventions to individual needs is crucial, considering the variability in psychological responses to dysphagia. Therapists work collaboratively with patients to develop coping mechanisms, resilience, and a positive mindset, mitigating the psychological impact of difficult swallowing on the overall quality of life.

In conclusion, the psychological effects of difficulty swallowing are multifaceted and require a customized, integrated approach. Healthcare providers can greatly enhance the overall quality of life for those who are managing their dysphagia by treating the psychological aspects of the condition.

Resources And Support Groups

Support groups and resources play a pivotal role in the comprehensive care and support system for individuals facing difficulty swallowing.

These groups serve as invaluable platforms for sharing experiences, exchanging information, and providing emotional support. Support groups may be facilitated by healthcare professionals, such as speech-language pathologists or psychologists, who guide discussions on coping strategies, adaptive techniques, and available resources.

The communal nature of these groups fosters a sense of belonging and understanding among participants, mitigating the isolation often associated with dysphagia. Additionally, online resources, including informative websites, virtual support groups, and educational materials, contribute to the dissemination of knowledge and support on a broader scale.

Integrating support groups and resources into the care plan empowers individuals with dysphagia, equipping them with the tools and knowledge to navigate the challenges they face.

Techniques Of Communication

Effective communication is a fundamental aspect of human interaction, and difficulty swallowing can significantly impact this essential skill. Individuals with dysphagia may encounter challenges related to speech clarity, voice quality, and overall communication effectiveness.

Speech-language pathologists play a crucial role in developing tailored communication strategies to address these challenges. This may involve exercises to enhance oral motor coordination, strategies to improve breath support for speech, and training on alternative communication methods, such as augmentative and alternative communication (AAC) devices.

Moreover, educating communication partners, including family members, friends, and caregivers, is essential to creating an inclusive and supportive environment. By implementing these communication strategies, individuals with difficult swallowing can maintain meaningful connections and actively participate in social interactions, mitigating the potential isolation associated with communication difficulties.

communication techniques are essential parts of the all-encompassing care model for people who have trouble swallowing. Resolving the communication issues related to dysphagia improves social interaction, builds mutual understanding in relationships, and raises quality of life in general.

Coping strategies, support groups, and communication strategies are interdependent components of the holistic care of people with dysphagia. Healthcare providers can improve the general health of people with dysphagia by addressing the psychological impact, establishing a supportive community through support groups, and putting into practice effective communication strategies.

This all-encompassing approach recognizes the multifaceted nature of dysphagia and stresses the significance of customized interventions that take into account the individual needs and experiences of each patient. As research and clinical practices continue to advance, more advancements in the comprehension and treatment of difficult swallowing are anticipated.

CHAPTER SEVEN
PREVENTION AND PROACTIVE CARE

Adopting A Healthier Lifestyle

Healthy lifestyle practices play a pivotal role in preventing difficult swallowing, also known as dysphagia. One of the fundamental aspects of maintaining a healthy lifestyle in this context is adequate hydration. Proper hydration ensures the lubrication of the throat, facilitating the smooth passage of food and liquids during swallowing. Dehydration can lead to dryness in the throat, making it difficult for the muscles involved in swallowing to function optimally.

Moreover, maintaining a balanced and nutritious diet is crucial. Consuming a variety of nutrient-rich foods supports overall health, including the muscles involved in the swallowing process. Malnutrition or deficiencies in key nutrients can contribute to muscle weakness, potentially leading to difficulties in swallowing.

Therefore, promoting and adhering to healthy lifestyle practices, such as staying adequately hydrated and maintaining a nutritious diet, can significantly contribute to the prevention of difficult swallowing.

Early Identification And Action

The best way to manage swallowing difficulties is to detect them early and take appropriate action. When swallowing difficulties are detected early, it is possible to address them and prevent further problems from arising. One way to do this is by regularly monitoring oneself for signs of dysphagia, such as persistent coughing during meals, feeling like food is stuck in the throat, or experiencing unexplained weight loss.

Healthcare professionals can also conduct assessments to identify swallowing difficulties in their early stages. Once swallowing difficulties are identified, appropriate interventions, such as dietary modifications, swallowing exercises, or medical treatments, can be put into action to address the underlying causes and improve swallowing function.

Frequent Examinations And Screenings

Regular medical examinations offer healthcare providers the chance to evaluate the patient's overall health, which includes the function of the swallowing mechanism.

Periodic screenings, which may involve imaging studies or diagnostic tests, allow for the early identification of potential risk factors or abnormalities that may lead to swallowing difficulties. These screenings may include video fluoroscopy, endoscopy, or other specialized tests to evaluate the anatomy and function of the throat and esophagus. In the context of difficult swallowing, regular check-ups and screenings are crucial components of proactive care. Additionally, they foster

CONCLUSION

difficult swallowing, or dysphagia, is a multifaceted condition that can significantly impact an individual's quality of life.

Prevention and proactive care are crucial aspects of managing and mitigating the challenges associated with swallowing difficulties. Healthy lifestyle practices, including proper hydration and balanced nutrition, serve as foundational elements in preventing dysphagia.

Adequate hydration ensures the optimal functioning of the muscles involved in swallowing, while proper nutrition supports overall muscle health. Early detection and intervention play a pivotal role in addressing swallowing difficulties before they escalate, allowing for targeted treatments and improved outcomes.

Regular check-ups and screenings further contribute to proactive care by facilitating the early identification of risk factors or abnormalities that may lead to dysphagia.

By embracing these preventive measures and incorporating them into healthcare routines, individuals can take proactive steps to maintain optimal swallowing function and enhance their overall well-being. Dysphagia, when addressed comprehensively through prevention and proactive care, can be managed effectively, leading to improved quality of life for those affected by this condition.